ROACCUTANE:

How to Guide

A Definitive Handbook on how Roaccutane is used to treat severe acne that hasn't responded to other treatments

Dr. Baker Rollins

Table of Contents

INTRODUCTION

PREFACE

Welcome to "Understanding Roaccutane: A Comprehensive Guide to Acne Treatment." This book is designed to provide an in-depth understanding of Roaccutane (also known as isotretinoin), one of the most effective treatments for severe acne. Whether you are a patient considering Roaccutane, a parent of a teenager struggling with acne, or a healthcare professional seeking detailed information, this book aims to serve as a valuable resource.

About This Book

Acne is more than just a skin condition; it can significantly impact one's self-esteem, emotional well-being, and overall quality of life. Roaccutane has been a game-changer for many individuals, offering relief when other treatments have failed. However, the decision to start Roaccutane treatment is not one to be taken lightly due to its potent effects and potential side effects. This book aims to provide a balanced view, covering both the benefits and the challenges associated with Roaccutane.

Understanding Acne: A Brief Overview

Before diving into the specifics of Roaccutane, it's important to understand acne itself. Acne is a common skin condition that affects millions of people worldwide. It occurs when hair follicles become clogged with oil and dead skin cells, leading to whiteheads, blackheads, pimples, and sometimes cystic lesions. While acne is most common among teenagers, it can persist or even start in adulthood.

Types of Acne

- **Comedonal Acne:** Characterized by whiteheads and blackheads.

- **Inflammatory Acne:** Involves red, swollen pimples.

- **Cystic Acne:** Severe form with deep, painful cysts and nodules.

Causes of Acne

- **Hormonal Changes:** Fluctuations in hormones, especially during puberty, menstruation, and pregnancy.

- **Genetics:** Family history can play a significant role.

- **Diet:** Certain foods may exacerbate acne in some individuals.

- **Stress:** Can trigger or worsen acne.

The Journey of Roaccutane

Roaccutane, a brand name for isotretinoin, has revolutionized the treatment of severe acne since its introduction. Developed in the 1980s, Roaccutane has provided hope for those who have not responded to other treatments. It works by reducing the size and output of sebaceous glands, normalizing skin cell turnover, and has anti-inflammatory properties. However, its powerful effects come with a range of potential side effects, necessitating careful consideration and medical supervision.

A Balanced Approach

This book aims to provide a thorough understanding of Roaccutane, addressing its history, scientific basis, treatment protocols, side effects, and impact on daily life. We also explore life after treatment, offering guidance on maintaining skin health and sharing personal stories from those who have undergone the treatment.

How to Use This Book

Each chapter is structured to give you detailed insights into different aspects of Roaccutane treatment:

- **Chapter 1** introduces Roaccutane, explaining its history, how it works, and who it is for.

- **Chapter 2** guides you through the treatment journey, from preparation and administration to managing side effects.

- **Chapter 3** discusses the impact of Roaccutane on daily life, including physical, mental, and lifestyle considerations.

- **Chapter 4** focuses on life after Roaccutane, offering tips for post-treatment care and reflecting on the journey.

Throughout the book, you'll find practical advice, scientific explanations, and real-life experiences to help you make informed decisions about Roaccutane treatment. Whether you are just starting to consider this medication or are already on your treatment journey, this book is designed to support you every step of the way.

Welcome to your comprehensive guide on Roaccutane. Let's embark on this journey together, towards clearer skin and improved well-being.

CHAPTER 1: UNDERSTANDING ROACCUTANE

1.1 THE HISTORY OF ROACCUTANE

Roaccutane, known generically as isotretinoin, was first introduced in the early 1980s. Developed by the pharmaceutical company Roche, it was initially created to treat certain types of cancer due to its potent ability to influence cell growth. However, its remarkable effectiveness in treating severe acne soon became apparent, leading to its approval by the FDA for acne treatment in 1982.

Key Milestones in Roaccutane's Journey

- **1982:** FDA approval for the treatment of severe recalcitrant nodular acne.

- **1990s:** Recognition of its potential side effects leads to increased scrutiny and regulatory measures.

- **2000s:** Implementation of stricter guidelines for prescription and usage, including pregnancy prevention programs due to teratogenic risks.

- **2010:** Generic versions become widely available, increasing accessibility and affordability.

1.2 The Science Behind Roaccutane

Roaccutane, a derivative of vitamin A, primarily works by reducing the size and activity of sebaceous glands, which produce the oil (sebum) that can clog pores and lead to acne. Additionally, it helps normalize skin cell turnover and possesses anti-inflammatory properties, reducing the formation of new acne lesions and promoting the healing of existing ones.

The Role of Isotretinoin

Isotretinoin is a retinoid, a class of compounds related to vitamin A. It exerts its effects by binding to nuclear receptors in the skin cells, influencing gene expression and modulating cellular differentiation and proliferation. This leads to a significant reduction in sebum production, changes in skin cell behavior, and anti-inflammatory effects, all of which contribute to its efficacy in treating severe acne.

1.3 Indications and Usage

Roaccutane is typically prescribed for individuals with severe recalcitrant nodular acne that has not responded to other treatments, including oral antibiotics and topical therapies. It is considered when:

- Acne causes significant psychological distress or physical scarring.

- Other treatments have failed to provide adequate results.

- The patient is capable of adhering to the strict guidelines, especially regarding pregnancy prevention for women of childbearing age.

Conditions Treated with Roaccutane

While primarily used for severe acne, Roaccutane has also been employed in treating other skin conditions and disorders, including:

- **Rosacea:** In cases where traditional treatments are ineffective.

- **Hidradenitis Suppurativa:** A chronic skin condition characterized by inflamed and swollen lumps.

- **Neuroblastoma:** As part of cancer treatment, due to its ability to influence cell differentiation.

Conclusion

Understanding the history, science, and appropriate usage of Roaccutane is crucial for those considering this powerful medication. Its development marked a significant advancement in dermatology, offering hope and relief to individuals struggling with severe acne. However, due to its potent effects and potential risks, it must be used under strict medical supervision with careful consideration of its indications and guidelines. In the next chapter, we will explore the treatment journey, including preparation, administration, and management of side effects.

CHAPTER 2: THE TREATMENT JOURNEY

2.1 PREPARING FOR ROACCUTANE TREATMENT

Before starting Roaccutane, a comprehensive medical evaluation is essential to ensure the safety and appropriateness of the treatment. This evaluation includes:

- **Medical History:** A thorough review of your medical history, including any past or current medical conditions, medications, and allergies.

- **Physical Examination:** A physical exam to assess the severity of acne and check for any underlying conditions that might contraindicate Roaccutane use.

- **Laboratory Tests:** Blood tests to check liver function, lipid levels, and a pregnancy test for women of childbearing age. These tests establish baselines and identify any potential issues that need monitoring during treatment.

Setting Realistic Expectations

Understanding what Roaccutane can and cannot do is crucial for a successful treatment journey. While Roaccutane is highly effective, results vary among individuals. It is important to:

- **Discuss Outcomes:** Have an open discussion with your healthcare provider about expected outcomes, potential side effects, and the duration of treatment.

- **Understand the Process:** Realize that initial worsening of acne is common before improvement is seen, usually within a few weeks to months.

- **Commitment to Follow-Up:** Be prepared for regular follow-up visits and ongoing laboratory tests to monitor progress and manage side effects.

2.2 The Course of Treatment

Roaccutane dosage is personalized based on weight, severity of acne, and response to treatment. General guidelines include:

- **Initial Dose:** Typically starts at 0.5 mg to 1 mg per kilogram of body weight per day.

- **Adjustments:** Dose adjustments based on tolerance and response, with a maximum dose of 2 mg/kg/day in severe cases.

- **Duration:** Treatment usually lasts 15 to 20 weeks, but some may require longer courses or additional cycles.

Monitoring Progress

Regular monitoring is essential to ensure the effectiveness and safety of Roaccutane treatment. This includes:

- **Monthly Check-Ups:** To evaluate skin improvement, side effects, and overall health.

- **Blood Tests:** Regular blood tests to monitor liver function, lipid levels, and for women, monthly pregnancy tests due to the high teratogenic risk.

- **Adherence to Guidelines:** Strict adherence to guidelines, especially for women of childbearing age who must use two forms of contraception and undergo monthly pregnancy tests.

2.3 Managing Side Effects

Roaccutane can cause a range of side effects, some of which are common and manageable:

- **Dry Skin and Lips:** Most common side effect, managed with moisturizers and lip balms.

- **Dry Eyes and Nose:** Use of artificial tears and nasal saline sprays can help.

- **Increased Sun Sensitivity:** Regular use of sunscreen and protective clothing.

Rare but Serious Side Effects

Some side effects are less common but require immediate medical attention:

- **Mental Health Changes:** Symptoms of depression, anxiety, or mood changes should be reported immediately.

- **Severe Skin Reactions:** Redness, blistering, or peeling skin requires urgent care.

- **Liver and Pancreas Issues:** Symptoms such as severe stomach pain, jaundice, or dark urine need prompt evaluation.

Coping Strategies

Effective management of side effects can enhance the treatment experience:

- **Stay Hydrated:** Drinking plenty of water to help manage dry skin.

- **Healthy Diet:** Eating a balanced diet to support overall health.

- **Support Systems:** Leaning on family, friends, or support groups for emotional support during treatment.

Starting Roaccutane treatment involves careful preparation, a structured treatment plan, and vigilant monitoring to manage side effects and ensure the best possible outcomes. Understanding the treatment process and being proactive in managing side effects can help make the journey smoother and more successful. In the next chapter, we will delve into the impact of Roaccutane on daily life, including physical, mental, and lifestyle considerations.

CHAPTER 3: IMPACT ON DAILY LIFE

3.1 PHYSICAL HEALTH CONSIDERATIONS

Roaccutane significantly affects the skin, necessitating a dedicated skin care regimen:

- **Moisturizers:** Regular use of non-comedogenic moisturizers helps combat dryness. Look for products containing ingredients like hyaluronic acid, ceramides, and glycerin.

- **Cleansers:** Gentle, hydrating cleansers that do not strip the skin of natural oils are essential. Avoid harsh soaps and exfoliants.

- **Lip Care:** Lips are particularly prone to dryness. Keep a lip balm with moisturizing ingredients like petroleum jelly or beeswax handy at all times.

Diet and Nutrition Tips

A balanced diet can support overall health and possibly enhance treatment outcomes:

- **Hydration:** Drink plenty of water to stay hydrated, aiding in managing dry skin and mucous membranes.

- **Healthy Fats:** Incorporate sources of healthy fats, such as avocados, nuts, and olive oil, which can help maintain skin elasticity.

- **Nutrient-Rich Foods:** Focus on a diet rich in vitamins and minerals, especially those beneficial for skin health, like vitamin E, zinc, and omega-3 fatty acids.

3.2 Mental and Emotional Well-being

Acne can have profound psychological effects, and starting Roaccutane may also come with emotional challenges:

- **Impact on Self-Esteem:** Severe acne can lead to decreased self-esteem and confidence. Understanding that Roaccutane can gradually improve skin can provide hope and motivation.

- **Mood Changes:** Be aware of potential mood changes associated with Roaccutane. Some patients report feelings of depression or anxiety. Regularly communicate with healthcare providers about any mental health changes.

Support Systems and Resources

Having a strong support network is crucial during treatment:

- **Family and Friends:** Lean on loved ones for encouragement and understanding.

- **Support Groups:** Join support groups, either in-person or online, to share experiences and gain advice from others undergoing similar treatment.

- **Professional Help:** Seek counseling or therapy if experiencing significant emotional distress. Mental health professionals can provide coping strategies and support.

3.3 Lifestyle Adjustments

Roaccutane increases sun sensitivity, making sun protection a critical part of daily life:

- **Sunscreen:** Use a broad-spectrum sunscreen with an SPF of 30 or higher. Apply generously and reapply every two hours when outdoors.

- **Protective Clothing:** Wear hats, sunglasses, and long sleeves to shield skin from the sun.

- **Avoid Tanning Beds:** Completely avoid tanning beds and intentional sun exposure.

Handling Physical Activities

Physical activities might require adjustments to avoid exacerbating side effects:

- **Hydration:** Ensure adequate hydration during and after exercise to manage dry skin.

- **Skin Protection:** Use gentle, non-irritating products post-exercise to clean sweat and bacteria from the skin.

- **Activity Choices:** Opt for lower-impact activities if experiencing joint or muscle discomfort, a possible side effect of Roaccutane.

Conclusion

The impact of Roaccutane on daily life extends beyond skin improvements. It involves careful attention to physical health, emotional well-being, and lifestyle adjustments. By adopting effective skin care routines, maintaining a balanced diet, managing emotional health, and protecting against sun exposure, patients can navigate the treatment journey more comfortably and successfully. In the next chapter, we will explore life after Roaccutane, including post-treatment skin care, personal reflections, and future perspectives on acne treatment.

CHAPTER 4: AFTER ROACCUTANE

4.1 POST-TREATMENT SKIN CARE

After completing a course of Roaccutane, maintaining the health of your skin is crucial to preserving the improvements and preventing new breakouts:

- **Continued Moisturization:** Continue using non-comedogenic moisturizers to keep your skin hydrated. Look for ingredients like ceramides and hyaluronic acid.

- **Gentle Cleansing:** Use mild, non-irritating cleansers to maintain skin barrier integrity. Avoid harsh scrubs and exfoliants.

- **Sun Protection:** Sunscreen remains essential. Use a broad-spectrum SPF 30 or higher daily to protect your skin from UV damage.

Long-term Skin Health Strategies

Long-term strategies help ensure your skin remains clear and healthy:

- **Regular Dermatologist Visits:** Periodic check-ups with your dermatologist can help monitor skin health and address any concerns early.

- **Topical Retinoids:** Your dermatologist might recommend continuing with topical retinoids to maintain results and prevent new acne.

- **Healthy Lifestyle:** Maintain a balanced diet, stay hydrated, and manage stress through regular exercise and mindfulness practices.

4.2 Reflecting on the Treatment

Reflecting on your journey with Roaccutane can be therapeutic and insightful:

- **Journaling:** Keep a journal to document your experience, noting the progress, challenges, and changes you've observed.

- **Before and After Photos:** Taking photos can help you appreciate the improvements and remind you of the progress made.

- **Sharing Your Story:** Consider sharing your experience in support groups or online forums to help others who are considering or currently undergoing treatment.

Lessons Learned

Reflecting on the lessons learned during your treatment can provide valuable insights:

- **Patience and Persistence:** Understand that significant improvements take time and persistence.

- **Self-Care Importance:** Recognize the importance of comprehensive self-care, including physical, emotional, and mental health aspects.

- **Support Systems:** Appreciate the role of a strong support network in managing and completing the treatment journey.

4.3 Future Perspectives

The landscape of acne treatment is continuously evolving with ongoing research and development:

- **New Medications:** Stay informed about new medications and treatments emerging in dermatology, such as biologics and novel topical therapies.

- **Technology and Procedures:** Advances in technology, like laser treatments and light therapies, offer additional options for acne management and scar reduction.

- **Personalized Medicine:** The future of acne treatment may lie in personalized medicine, tailoring treatments based on individual genetic and microbiome profiles.

The Evolving Landscape of Dermatological Care

Dermatological care continues to advance, with a growing emphasis on holistic and patient-centered approaches:

- **Integrative Approaches:** Combining traditional treatments with complementary therapies, such as dietary modifications and stress management techniques.

- **Teledermatology:** Increased access to dermatological care through telemedicine, allowing for convenient consultations and follow-ups.

- **Patient Education:** Ongoing education and empowerment of patients to make informed decisions about their skin health.

Life after Roaccutane involves continued care and vigilance to maintain the benefits achieved during treatment. By adopting effective skin care routines, staying informed about new treatment options, and reflecting on the personal journey, individuals can enjoy long-lasting results and improved skin health. This chapter concludes our comprehensive guide on Roaccutane, offering insights into each stage of the treatment journey, from understanding and preparation to daily life impact and post-treatment care. Remember, achieving clear and healthy skin is a continuous journey, and with the right knowledge and support, it is entirely attainable.

THE END